Learn How to
Run Faster Easily

2021 Edition

Table of Contents

BELLE & WINSLEY PRESS

How You Can Run Faster Effortlessly
By Adam D'Alessandro
First Edition, 2013

Introduction

14 years ago, I decided to compete in a half marathon. Having a month or so to prepare, I thought I'd start running on the local oval track just to see how I would fare against some of the locals.

It didn't take long for me to realize how slow I was running, as hordes of runners passed me several times on the oval track. Now I knew I wasn't the fastest guy on the track but having hordes of runners pass me by before I could finish running a couple of rounds of 400 meters was ridiculous!

Fast forward a month when I joined the half marathon and that's when I realized I was finishing the marathon near the last batch of guys my age. About the only group of guys who were behind me were the ones who were walking and too exhausted to finish the marathon.

Like most guys, I was frustrated. I ended up blaming genetics and my lack of athleticism for my embarrassing finish. Of course it's always mom and dad's fault!

Weeks passed by and I still couldn't stand the thought of finishing near dead last so I thought to myself "I've had it!!!" I'm going buy some books, videos and do whatever it takes to learn this stuff.

Why I made this book?

For the next few years, I had been searching for ways to become a faster runner. And what I've often seen are running plans and trite advice such as:

"Shoot for 9 to 12 miles a week."

"If you run a certain number of miles, ¼ of those should be quality miles."

The traditional way of looking at someone who's fast at running is to look at one or a combination of these:

- Length of their legs
- The number of hours or miles per session
- The ratio of junk miles per session
- How many months/years they've been training
- The length of their steps
- Their level of cardiovascular fitness
- The amount of effort/willpower they have

I asked myself what if there is a way for anyone to run faster regardless of age, level of cardiovascular fitness, effort, or "superior" genetics because of longer legs.

It wasn't until 12 years ago that some of the Kenyans started dominating the local running scene. They snagged the 1st, 2nd and 3rd places, shutting out everyone.

Taking heed from an old Arab proverb "Ask the experienced rather than the learned!" I started observing how they ran in the local track. One of the Kenyans that I observed was Joma, a guy in his late forties.

Now I can tell you this guy looked very normal. He didn't have long limbs that most of the fast runners have. He wasn't particularly explosive either when I watched him run, but he was fast!

I didn't expect a guy his age to keep up with the best local Kenyan runners for more than a 400-meter round at the track but there he was. The guy was keeping up with the best local Kenyan runners for several rounds.

What struck me though was that his face seemed relaxed throughout the run. It almost seemed as if he moved with near-effortless speed. He looked more like he was gliding through the whole thing.

That was when I decided to observe what separates the great runners from the rest of the pack. Throughout my years of coaching, I've seen runners of different ages, shapes and sizes and the one thing that great runners have in common is having the proper running form.

What are some of the bio-mechanics involved in running faster and how can someone achieve that kind of speed easily?

In this book, you'll find the answers to those questions as well as the secrets that the best Kenyan runners have that enables them to run faster and effortlessly. I hope you'll enjoy learning some of the techniques and principles of running as much as I do in teaching them.

Overview

The first part of this book teaches you how to have correct form in the torso area and how it helps your running. Use the drills shown at the end of the chapter to improve the form of your upper body.

The second part of the book shows you the proper mechanics for your legs and feet. It also shows you why it's important to have them. At the end of each chapter, use the drills to improve your mechanics. You also have the different kinds of stretches that you can incorporate in your warm-up and stretch routine that can significantly help with your stride.

The third part of the book tackles proper breathing and why it's crucial for you to breathe properly when running. The fourth part of the book details additional stretches and drills to help your alignment when running. The last part of the book tackles most of the frequently asked questions about running.

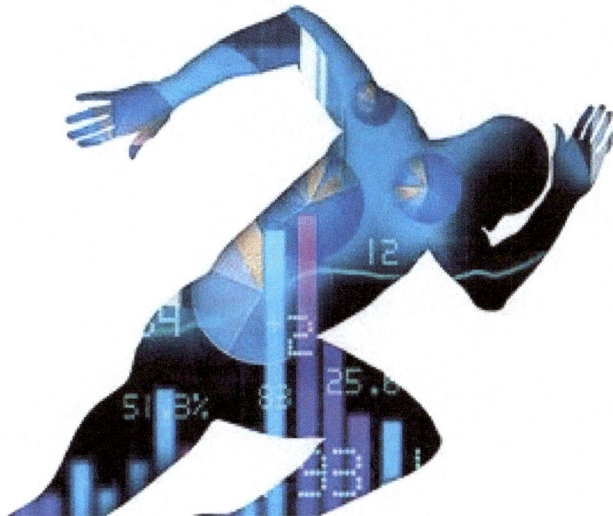

How to use this book:

Most of the time trying to improve your running form is as much about unlearning as it is about learning.

Try to incorporate one or two techniques at a time and keep in mind that your running form improves as your muscle memory of getting the right repetition improves.

Adding and perfecting some of the techniques in this book will vary from one person to another. Some techniques can take only a few minutes to master while others can take months. I suggest you try the one that's easiest for you and gives you the most in terms of results.

While you're at it, take note of **how performing the correct technique feels.** This is called *kinesthetic awareness* and it is one of the most important things you can learn from this book. **Knowing how to perform the correct technique intellectually and actually having the muscle memory to perform it are two different things.** Try to do these techniques slowly at first so you can get a feel for the movement. You can gradually increase the speed as you get better at it.

Here's a list of things that beginners struggle with:
- Being able to run faster
- Being able to run effortlessly
- Sustaining their ideal speed when running
- Getting more distance in their runs
- Avoiding injuries

All of these can be corrected by teaching principles and techniques of efficient running form.

Although these techniques may look like minor changes in your running form, you'll notice how the subtle differences can quickly add up to give you a lot of advantages.

The secret that the best runners have is efficiency. Most of the time they expend very little energy to achieve and sustain their ideal speed.

General Principles & Ideas To Maximize Your Speed.

Your genetics are not the reason why you're slow. Far too often, you'll hear beginners incessantly blaming their genetics for their slow speed. They'll probably blame everything on the length of their lower limbs, the lack of fast twitch muscle fibers, the ratio of the length of one limb to another or the simple fact that they have flat feet.

It is natural for most beginners to point to their genetics. After all, genetics really do affect how they run. The problem comes when people develop an attitude of learned helplessness and believe that there is nothing they could do to improve their running speed.

Nothing could be further from the truth. I've seen some of the fastest runners, who have shorter legs.

What separates the guys who run with effortless speed from those who struggle at running faster and improving their endurance?

In a word, it's having excellent running form. I cannot emphasize this enough because no aspect of running is as important, effective and efficient at giving your drastic and effortless improvements in speed.

What some beginners don't realize is that our bodies are built to run. You may not be an elite athlete but you can be a great runner. And I'm willing to bet that most of the guys have not maximized their potential to run faster. In the end, it's what you do with what you've got that makes all the difference.

Here are some of the principles and general ideas that you need to keep in mind when running:

Keep everything close to your center of gravity.

This principle encompasses a lot of the techniques that will be discussed in this book. The center of gravity is mostly located in our hips. In running, we want our center of gravity (COG) to travel in a horizontal line as much as possible.

Energy that is spent moving your COG up and down is wasted energy.

Most beginners try to take unnaturally long strides and overextend their bodies. This results in their COG moving up and down too much.

Moving your limbs too far away from your center of gravity also results in mechanical inefficiencies that result in wasted energy.

In the latter chapters, you'll see why it's important to keep everything compact and close to your COG.

Minimize the waste of energy.

The energy used by our body must be maximized by eliminating unnecessary movements that don't contribute to your body's forward movement such as unnecessary twisting of the body and creating longer lever arms.

Moreover, the use of bigger muscles over smaller muscles in generating power must be emphasized in order to sustain your ideal speed.

Chapter 1

The Importance of Your Torso

What easily distinguishes novice runners from good runners is the way they move their arms and torso. I'm sure you've seen a lot of action movies where you see someone running. More often than not you'll see them swing their arms across their upper body and twisting their upper torso.

Running this way seems natural. In fact, you'll often see this kind of movement in different spots such as football and basketball.

The problem comes when people look at this as the right way to run marathons or sprints. Football and basketball players often run this way because they need to able to stop, change directions or move laterally in an instant. When it comes to running, moving your arms across your torso, doesn't contribute to locomotion- the forward movement of your body.

While, it's one of the easiest to correct, most novice runners will insist on doing it that way too because they "feel faster." But twisting your torso doesn't help you move forward at all.

Mistake #1 Swinging your arms across the center of your torso

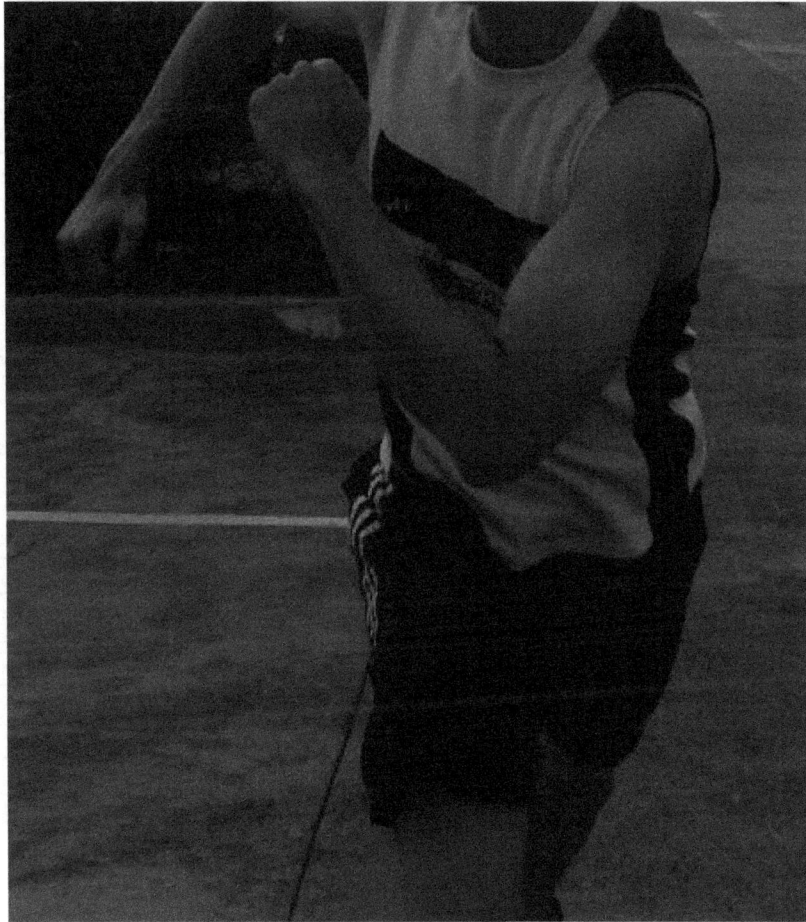

Fig. 1A Notice how his torso twists as it follows his arms across the centerline?

Instead of doing this, try to prevent your torso from twisting, by not letting your arms cross the torso and not having your hands swing behind the ears and elbows as shown in the pictures below:

Technique #1 Keep your arms on your sides when swinging your arms.

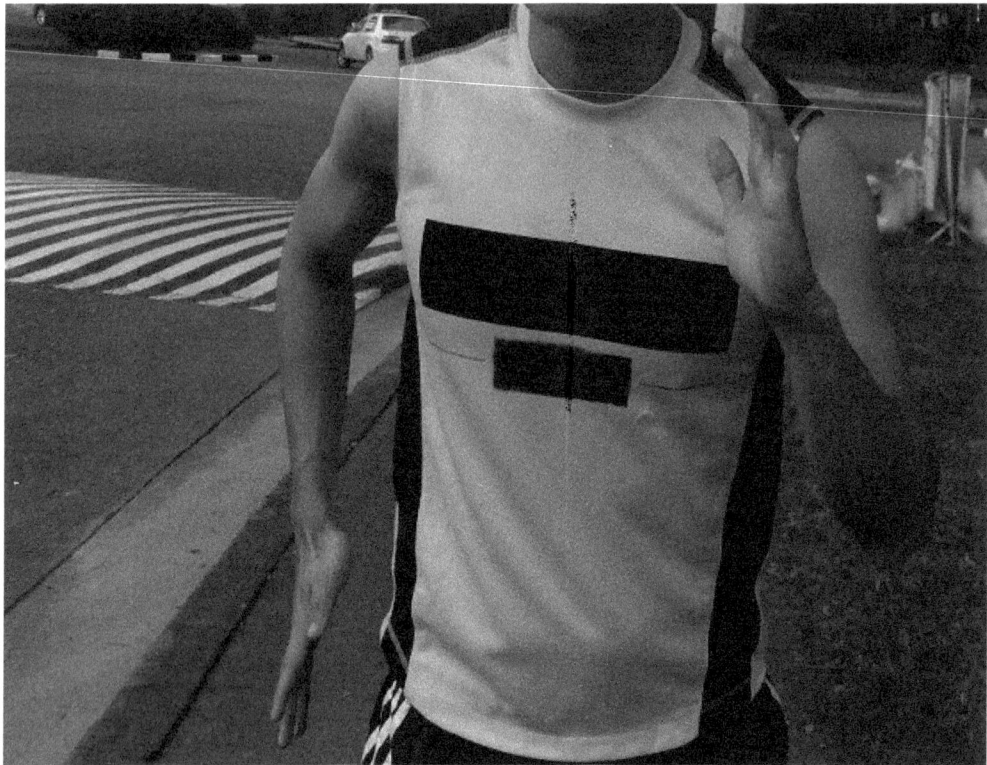

Fig. 1C Now, look at the proper way to swing the arms,
there is no wasted energy with the torso not twisting unnecessarily.

Technique #2 When swinging your arms, your hands should not pass the ears and pockets. Have approximately a 90 degree angle on the elbows.

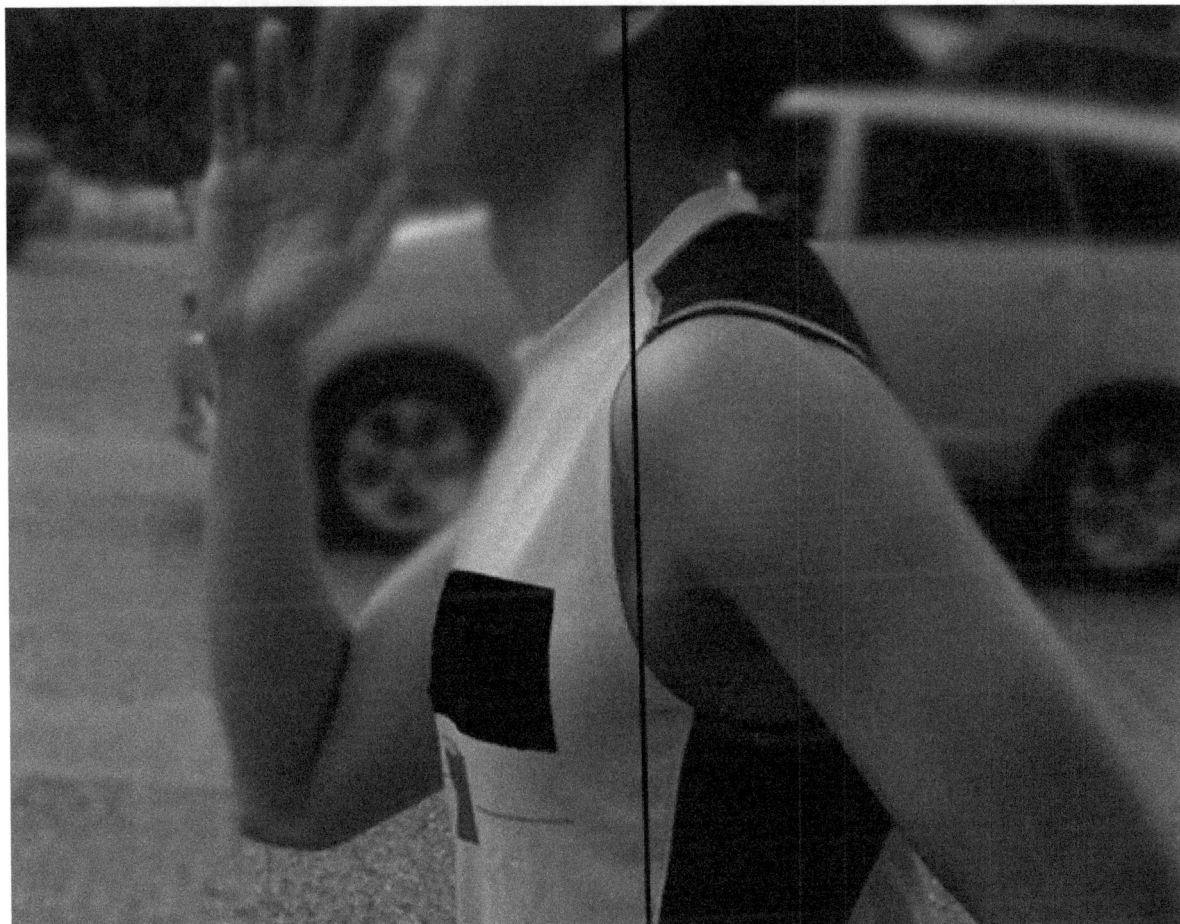

Fig. 1D If you can imagine a line from his ears down to his pocket below the hands should not go past that line. Only the elbows can move past the line.

Another favorite of novice runners is slouching, rounding their backs and raising their shoulders as they breathe when running. Now I'll admit I used to slouch a lot when I started running.

I remember one running coach telling me:
"And you're slouching like this. How can you breathe?"

I objected "but I feel faster."

He shot back "You think you're going faster because you're struggling for breath!"

Mistake # 2 Slouching , raising & rounding your shoulders forward when running

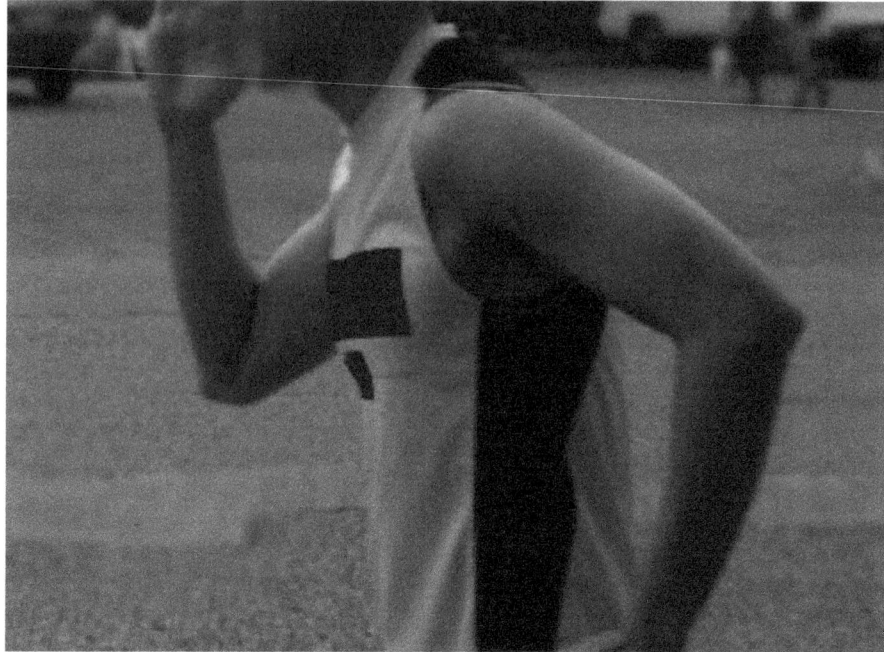

Fig. 1B Most runners get this kind of posture near the end of the race. Notice how difficult it is for him to breathe this way.

Technique #3 Keep your torso upright while keeping your shoulders down & relaxed.

Why is it important to keep an upright torso?
- You waste less energy because your back muscles won't keep on compensating as it keeps your body erect while running.

- It helps you breathe better.

Keep in mind that your body will be leaning forward slightly throughout the run however you will need to keep the alignment of your heard shoulders, and hips throughout.

Arm Circles Drill

Here's a drill that will help you keep your shoulders from rounding forward.

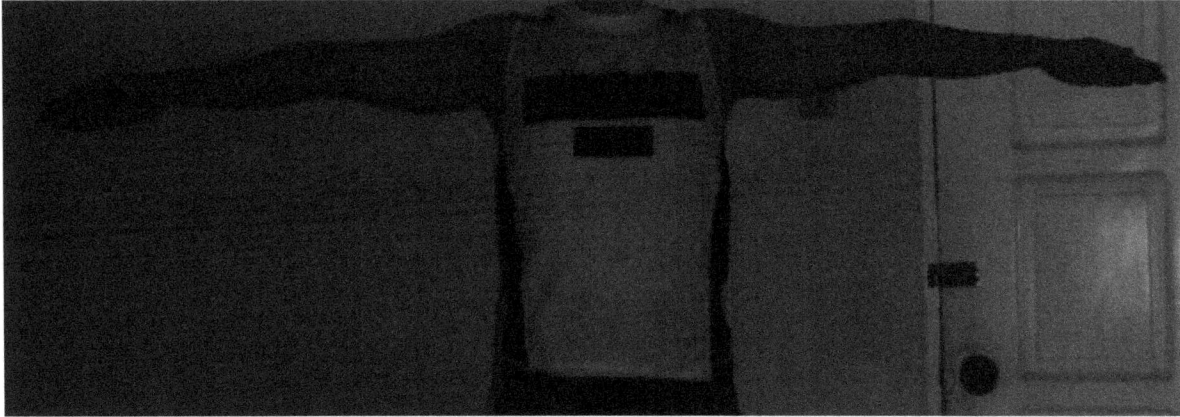

Fig. 1 E Remember that as you're doing this, you want to keep your shoulders down and relaxed as much as possible.

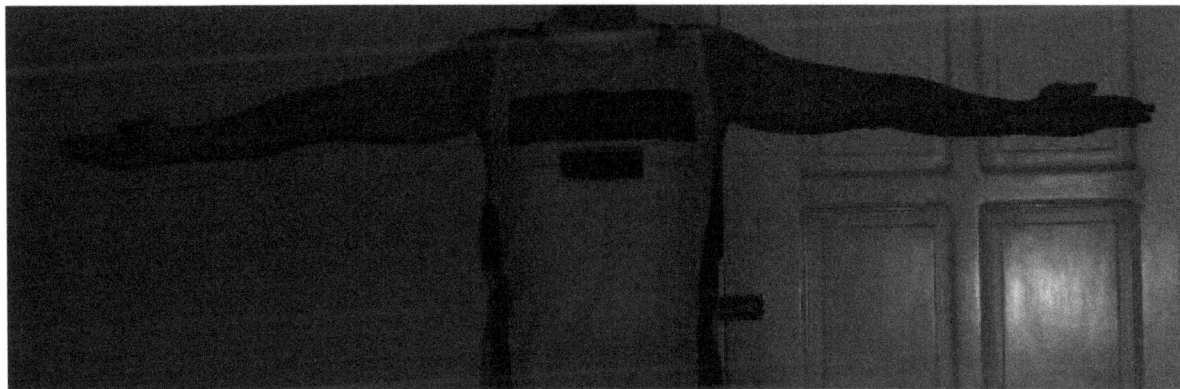

Fig. 1F

1.) Spread your arms to the sides as shown on fig. 1E.
2.) Make forward circles with your arms and feel your shoulder blades pinch together.
3.) Do this for 30 seconds to a minute.
4.) Now have your palms face up as shown in Fig. 1F and make reverse circles and once again feel the shoulder blades as they pinch together.
5.) Do this for 30 seconds to a minute.

Chapter 2

Adding More Speed Through Efficiency

One of the biggest things that I've observed with the best runners usually happens during the swing phase- the part when the foot comes off the ground and swings forward. The great runners often raise their knees a bit higher than most runners during the swing phase while most beginners don't raise their knees enough.

I can still remember a week of watching Joma coach some teenagers when I started running.

"Raise those knees some more!!!" he said.
" but it's exhausting."the other kid replied.
"Raise your knees!"

I couldn't figure out why he wanted them to raise their knees forward when I thought they were doing just fine. At that time I'm pretty sure the kids were thinking the same thing.

It wasn't until a few years after that I figured it out as I got a hold of some videos & started watching them in slow motion. A couple of hours of watching and I noticed the same thing over and over again: They were raising their knees higher than most beginning runners.

I discovered that what they were doing was simple physics! The lower limbs act as a lever and by raising the knees, they were effectively shortening the lever arm. Doing this requires less force to swing the leg forward.

Technique #4 Raise your knees forward to shorten your limb length as it swings forward during swing phase.

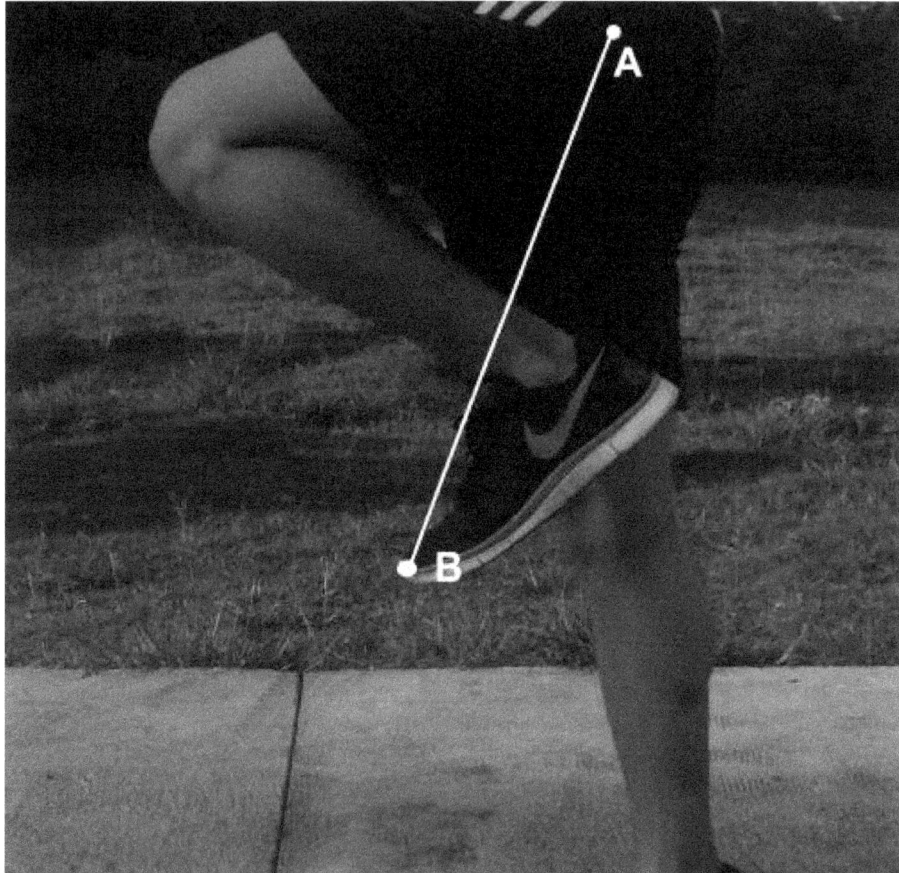

Fig. 2A When you raise your knees you effectively shorten the lever arm from point A to B.Compare this to Fig. 2B.

Here's what happens when you don't raise your knees. You end up lengthening the lever arm, which results in mechanical inefficiency.

Mistake #3 Not raising your knees and shortening the length of the limbs

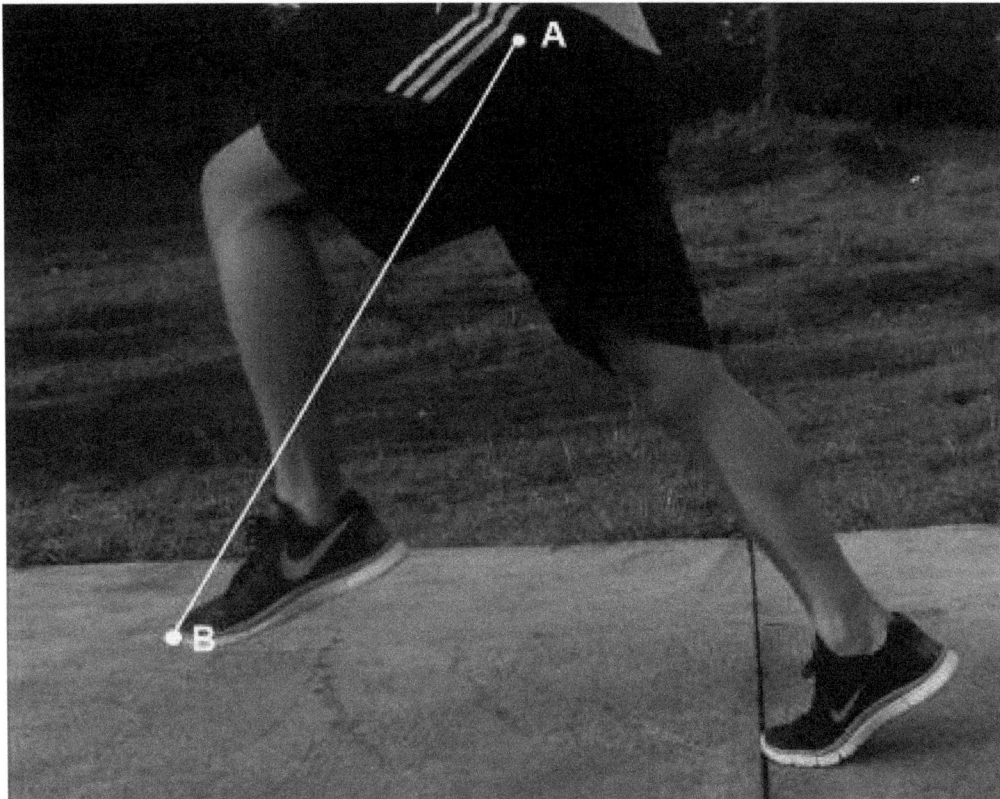

Fig. 2B The longer the lever arm , the more effort
you'll have to exert when running.

Notice also that as you raise your knees, your ankles are close to and aligned with your COG, This serves to prevent you from creating any kind of back-drag, which we'll discuss later.

Here's a drill that you can use to practice this technique.

One Foot Jump Drill
1.) Jump off of one foot while raising your knees on the other leg.
2.) Do this for 30 seconds to a minute on each leg.

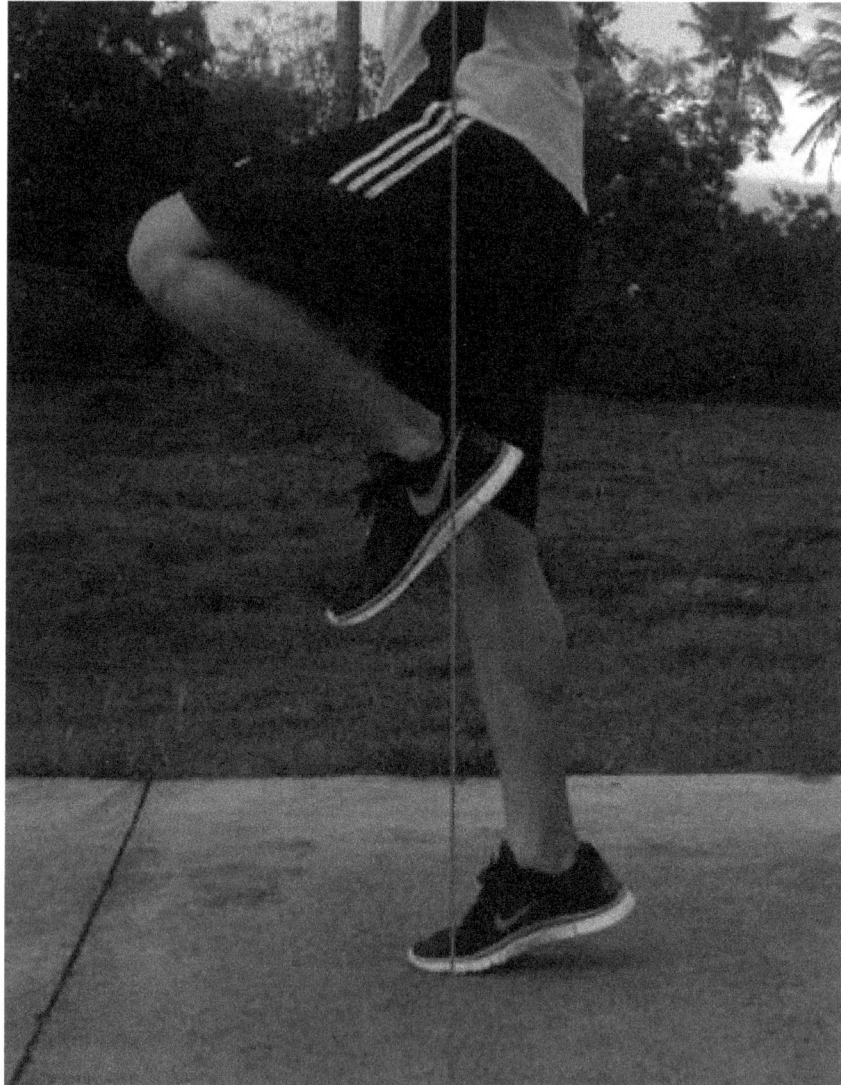

*You're doing it right if your ankle lines up
with your COG as shown in the picture.*

Chapter 3

The Key To Increasing Your Speed

A lot of beginners often ask me how they can run without getting tired after a few miles.

For some reason they think there's something wrong with their endurance but what I found out is that almost all of them are running on their heels.

Now here's what I want you to try out for yourself:
Try running a few meters on your heels without letting the forefoot or the balls of your feet touch the ground. Do you notice how goofy and awkward that feels? It won't take more than few minutes of running on your heels to realize that it's a recipe for disaster on your lower limbs.

Notice how it's nearly impossible to generate any kind of power from your legs? Do you notice that only your knees and hips are generating the power for you to run? And even then your knees can't even generate that much power at all.

Most beginners land on their heels during footstrike, a phase when your foot touches the ground. This creates a stopping motion. What ends up happening is similar to driving a car while stepping on the gas and breaks at the same time. Imagine how much energy is wasted!

The heels are meant to be used mainly for stability & stopping. When you look at a game where there's a lot of running, changing directions and stopping like basketball, you'll notice it. Look at how basketball players use their heels to stop as they get close to the ring to shoot the ball.

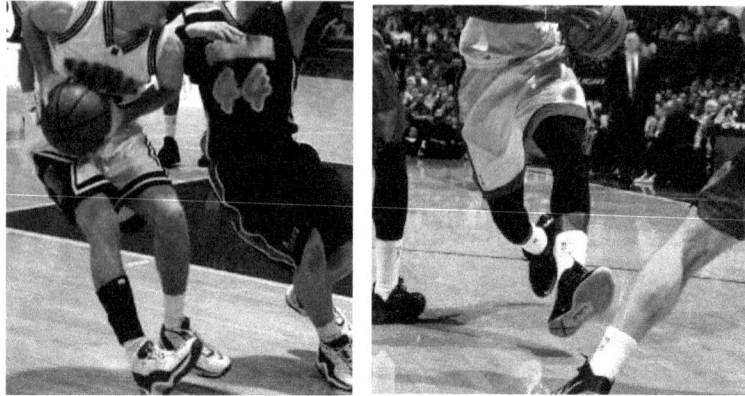

Fig. 3A & B Notice how the players lands with their heels first as they stop and bring the ball up to shoot?

The same thing happens every time you use your heels to land when you run.

Notice also that there's a lag time as your heels strikes the ground and transfers your weight from the heels to the ball of foot before your foot moves off the ground again.

Mistake #4 Using your heels to strike the ground

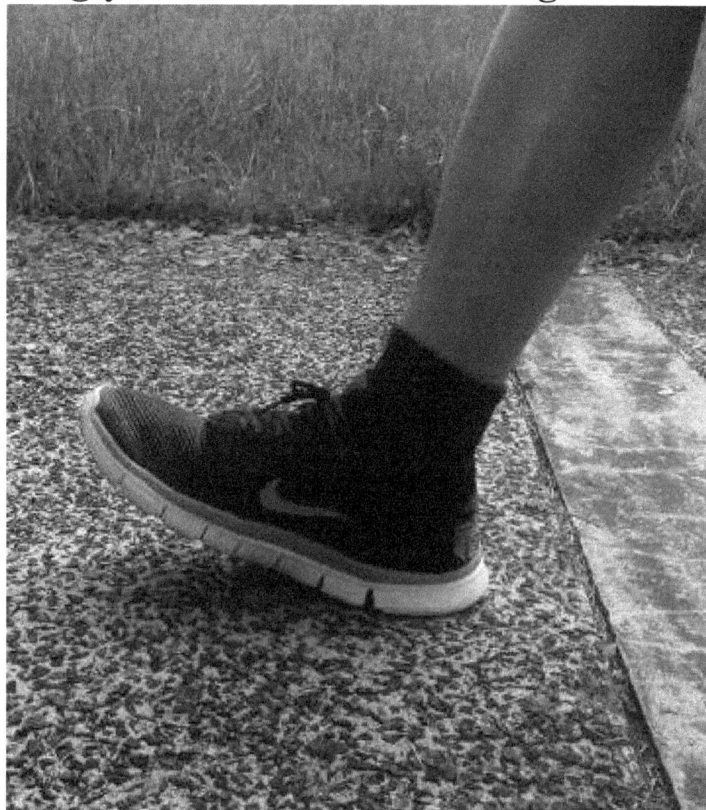

Fig. 3C When you use your heels to land on the ground, you're basically creating a stopping motion over and over again and making yourself very prone to injury.

So what part of the foot lands during footstrike?

If you answered your forefoot or the balls of your feet, you got it right.

So why land on the balls of your feet?
Here are some of the advantages:

- You're able to generate more power with more levers at work. *See the illustration below*

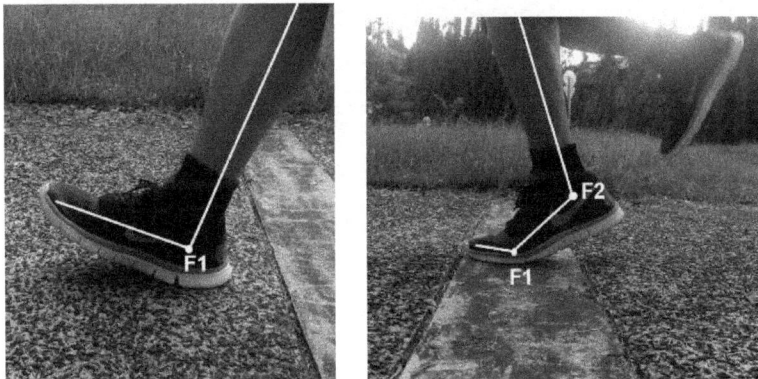

- The balls of your feet will act like a powerful spring as it strikes the ground.
- You're less susceptible to knee injuries and shin splints.

Technique #5 Land on the ball of your foot/forefoot during footstrike

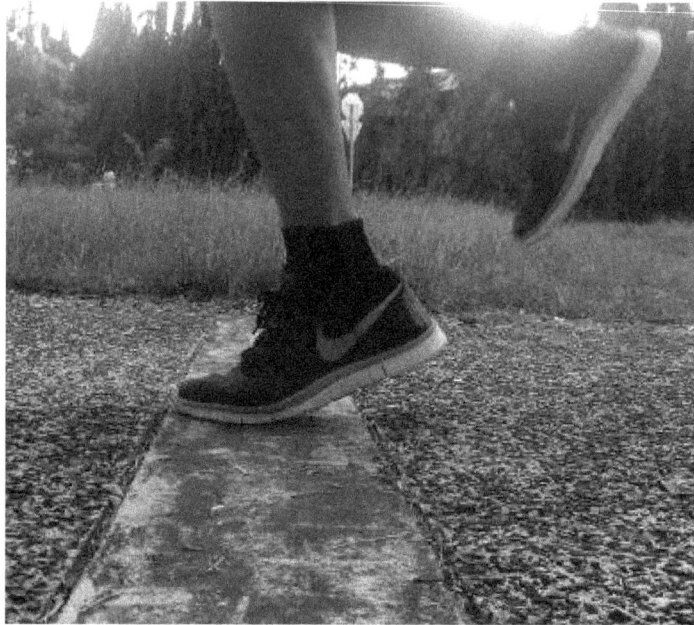

One of the most well-respected running coaches, Nicholas Romanov gives an analogy of using the ball of the foot as mimicking the structure of the legs of the fastest animals.[1] See the picture on the next page:

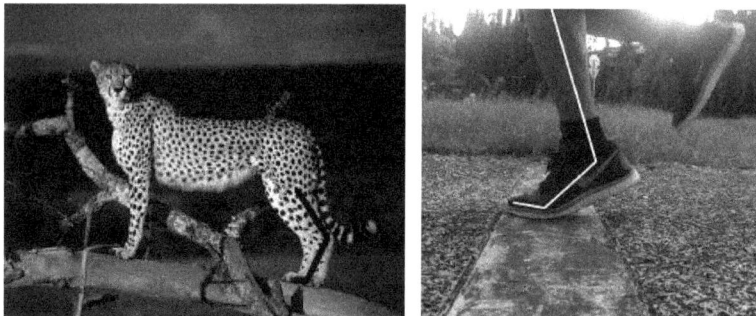

Fig. 3C & 3D Having this kind of structure creates an explosiveness in your step.

By now, I hope I've convinced you that landing on the balls of your feet is so much better. It is one of the keys to making you a faster runner.

Drill #4
Here are some drills that can help you land on the balls of your feet:

    1.)Uphill running
I usually recommend using uphill running as a way for some of the worst heel strikers to get a feel for using the balls of their feet. On steeper surfaces, it's impossible for their heels to touch the ground.
    2.)Skipping Rope
It's almost impossible to create any kind of rhythm skipping rope on your heels.
Note: You can do without the rope first, if you're not used to it. Just make sure you skip off the balls of your feet.

1. Ish Ledesma, dir. The POSE Method of Running. Perfs. Dr. Nicholas Romanov. Ish Ledesma, 2001.

Chapter 4

Components of Speed

If you've ever watched a 200-meter race on television, you'll often hear analysts give their comments about an athlete's stride length (the length of each step). They'll often rave about how a certain athlete has some kind of unfair advantage because of it and to a certain extent it's true. Having a great stride length is indeed an advantage.

So what do most beginners do? They overstride by taking steps that are unnaturally long. As a result, they get exhausted faster than they could imagine because having any kind of exaggerated stride is not sustainable for anybody.

They don't realize that having a long stride is only half of the equation. Speed is a product of the length of your stride and the frequency of the stride.

The equation goes like this:
Speed= length of your steps x frequency of your steps

Mistake #5 Taking strides that are unnaturally long

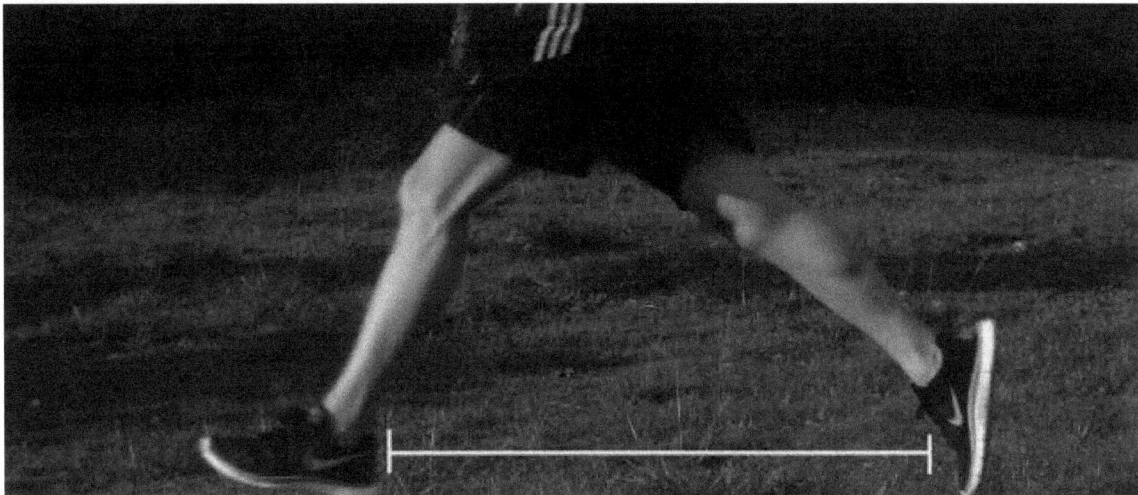

Figure 4A Look at how the lower limbs on the right leg is so far out of the center of gravity.

Increasing your speed is a delicate balance between the length of your steps and the frequency of your steps. Being able to balance both for optimal results is one of the most important factors when it comes to running faster with ease.

You can benefit more from trying to shorten your steps while increasing the frequency of steps. This not only enables you to achieve your optimal speed but to sustain it as well.

Technique #6 Shorten the length of your stride and increase the frequency of your steps

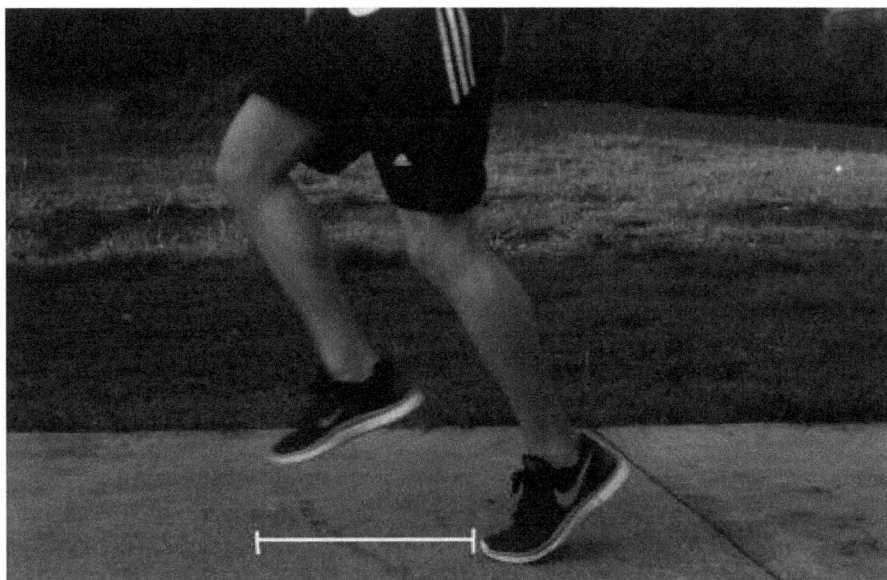

Why is it more sustainable? Here are a few reasons:

- If you'll recall the principles we discussed earlier, the closer your limbs are to your center of gravity the shorter the lever arm, which results in less effort for your body.
- More importantly, you end up not running on your heels and exposing yourself to injury.
- You run on the balls of your feet, which gives you more explosiveness.

How your arms affect stride frequency

One of the most hotly debated topics in running is the role of the arms. Some coaches say the arms are only there for stability and balance. Some would argue that pumping your arms increases your speed.

I believe in the latter. Pumping your arms faster enables you to increase your stride frequency and allows you to run faster.

Technique #7 Faster arm swing helps you increase your stride frequency.

Bonus Chapter 4.1

The Secrets of Elite Kenyan Runners: How to Increase Your Stride Length Naturally

Remember when I said that one of the main components of speed is stride length and how you shouldn't exaggerate the length of your stride by overstriding? Now you're probably asking what the difference is between overstriding and improving your natural stride. Here's one of the biggest secrets that I've seen from the Kenyan runners that will help you increase your speed tremendously.

Imagine both of your legs as part of an angle. **The greater that angle becomes, the longer your stride length becomes**. This helps you cover more ground without overextending your lower legs and creating an overstride angle as shown in the figure below. This is the angle of your natural stride or the angle of your hip extension. Improving your range of motion in this area is the key to becoming an excellent runner. Compare the figures below:

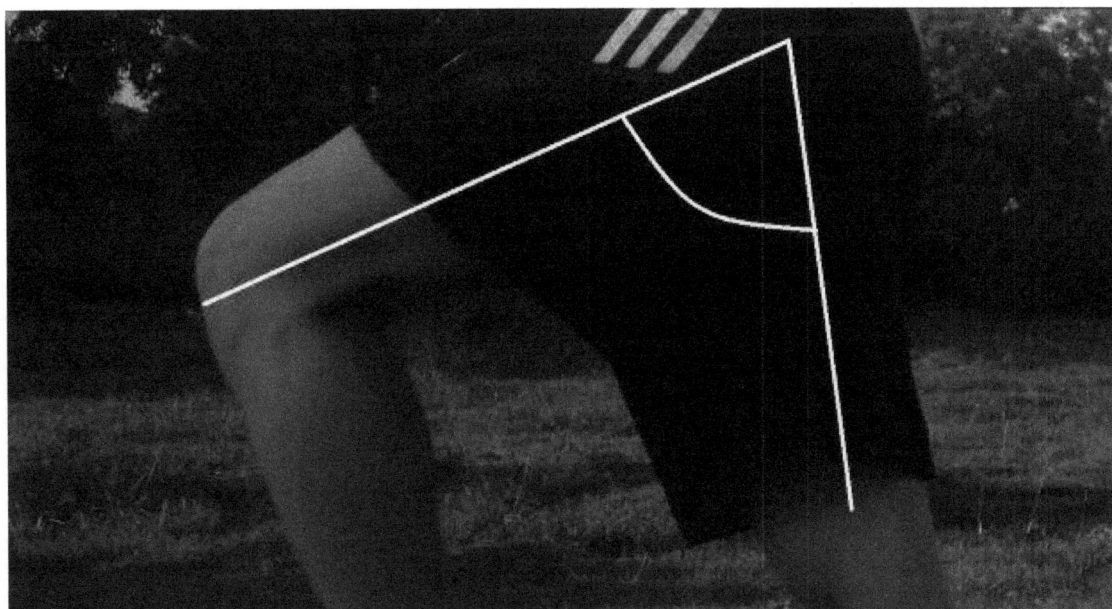

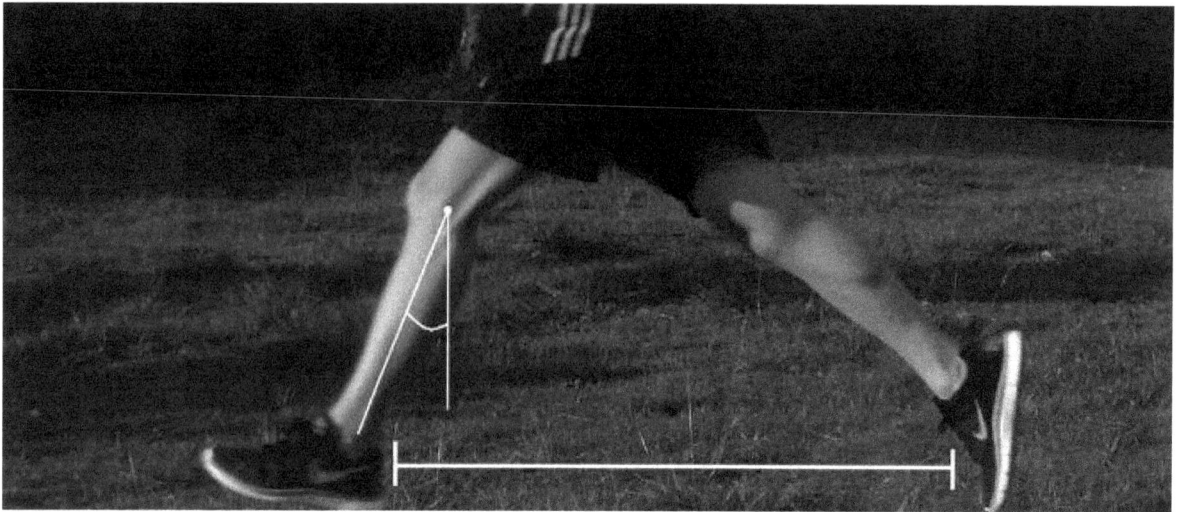

Figure 4D Notice the angle shown in the picture. That is the angle of the overstride. Runners should avoid this and strive to have a negative angle where the lower leg does not move past the knee.

Technique #8
Increase your stride length by increasing the angle of your natural stride while having a negative overstride angle.

I cannot emphasize the importance of this technique enough. The difference in executing this technique is what separates the elite runners from the rest of the pack. Find the time to do these stretches before your runs for a minimum of 3 times per week.

Kneeling Lunge Stretch
1.) Kneel on one leg
2.) Make sure your hips and limbs are aligned
3.) Slowly slide the foot of the other leg forward as your hips sink downward
4.) Make sure you don't lean forward and keep your toes in front of your knees.

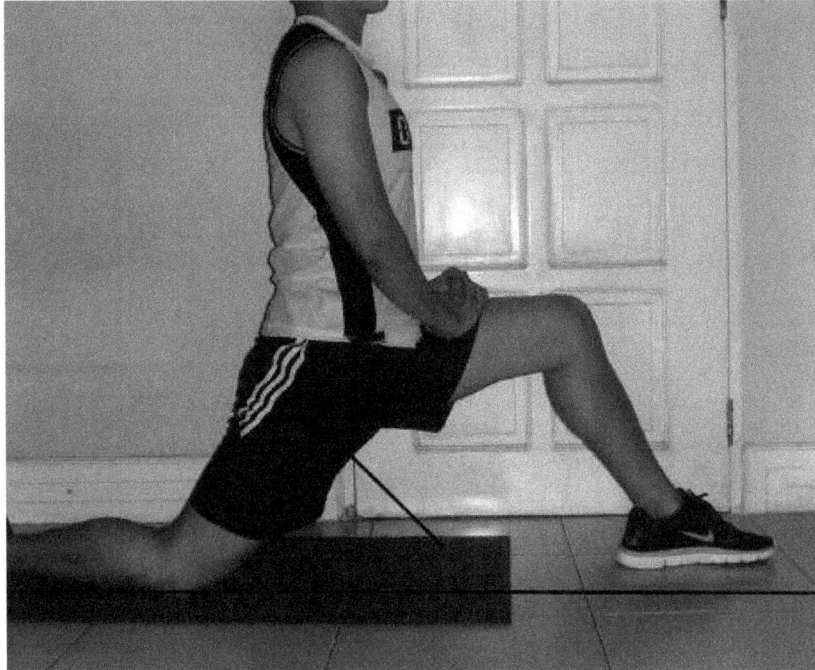

The arrow points to the part where you should

be feeling the stretch. Your legs, feet and hips
should be parallel to the horizontal line
as shown in the picture.

5.) Hold this stretch for 30 seconds to a minute and a half.
6.) Slowly sink your hips downward as you get better at this exercise

Assisted Runner's Stretch

The main goal of this stretch is to increase the flexibility of your hamstring muscles to improve the range of your upper legs as it swings on your lower hip.[2]

1.) Start kneeling on one knee and have it touch and stay in line with the back of the other foot. Let your hands rest on a chair or any object. See the picture below.

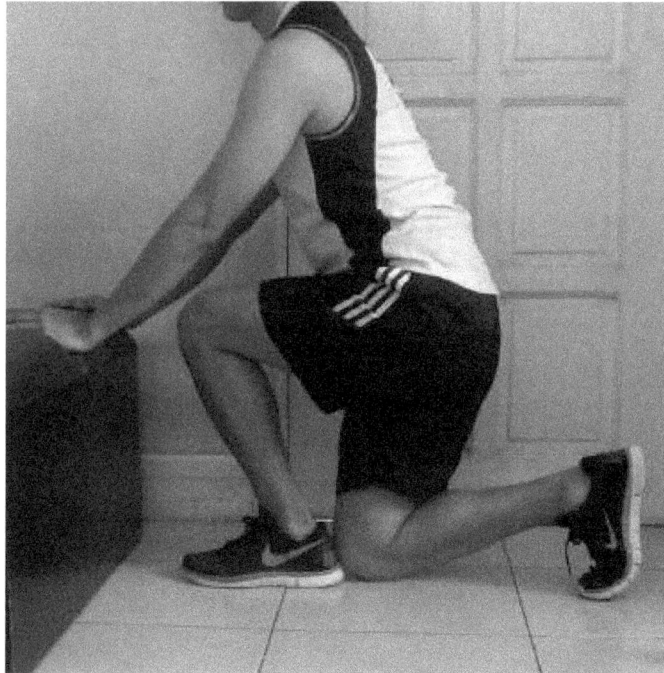

2.) With your hands rested on the object, slowly stand up and stretch the hamstring muscles of both legs as shown in the picture.

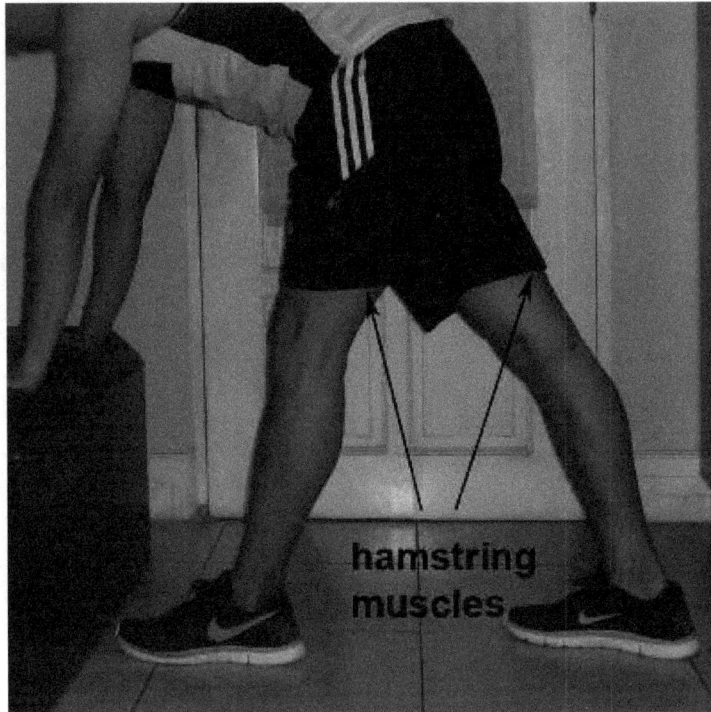

Remember to keep both legs straight.
If you need to, you can increase the height of
the chair or the object.

3.) You should be able to feel your hamstring muscles stretching.

4.) Hips should be level and you don't want it tweaking out to one side to compensate for the difficulty of the stretch.

5.) Also remember to keep all parts of both feet flat on the ground. Most people tend to roll either or both feet to one side to compensate.

6.) Hold it for a minute and a half. The goal is to reach 2 minutes.

7.) Alternate the legs and do it for the other side.

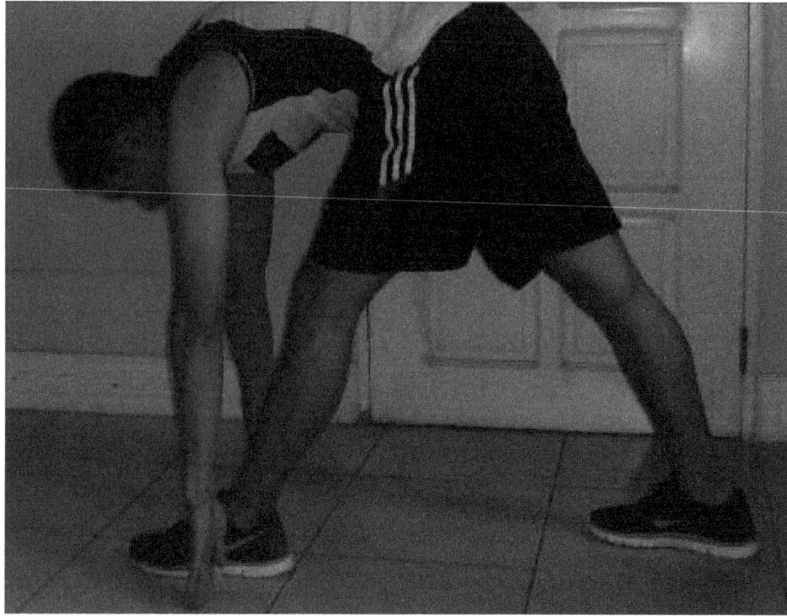

*Eventually, you should be able to touch the
ground and hold the stretch for the same
amount of time. Do this for both sides.*

8.) Remember to breathe deeply as well. Most novice runners hold their breath when performing this stretch.

Here's a stretch that was shown by Joanna Zeiger, an Olympic athlete that helps you open up your stride.[3]

Quadricep Stretch

The main goal of this exercise is to stretch the psoas and the quadriceps muscle. These are the muscles on the front of your upper leg.

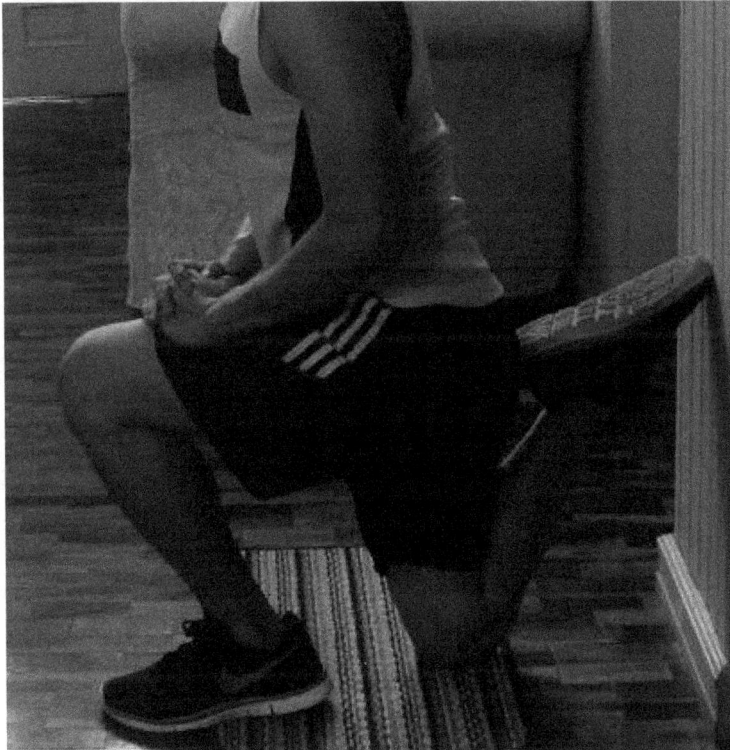

1.) Keep your back straight and kneel on one leg with your toes touching the wall.

2.) Keep your foot and your knees pointed straight ahead. Do not turn your knees inward.

3.) Hold this stretch for a minute and a half.

4.) If you squeeze the glutes (butt muscles) you'll feel it more on the stretch.

5.) The eventual goal is to get the knee of the kneeling leg as close to the wall as possible.

6.) Alternate the legs and do this for the other side.

IT Band Stretch

This exercise helps you stretch your ilio-tibial band.[4]

1.) Lie flat on your back with a 90 degree angle on yout hips and knees.
2.) Cross your legs as shown in the picture below:

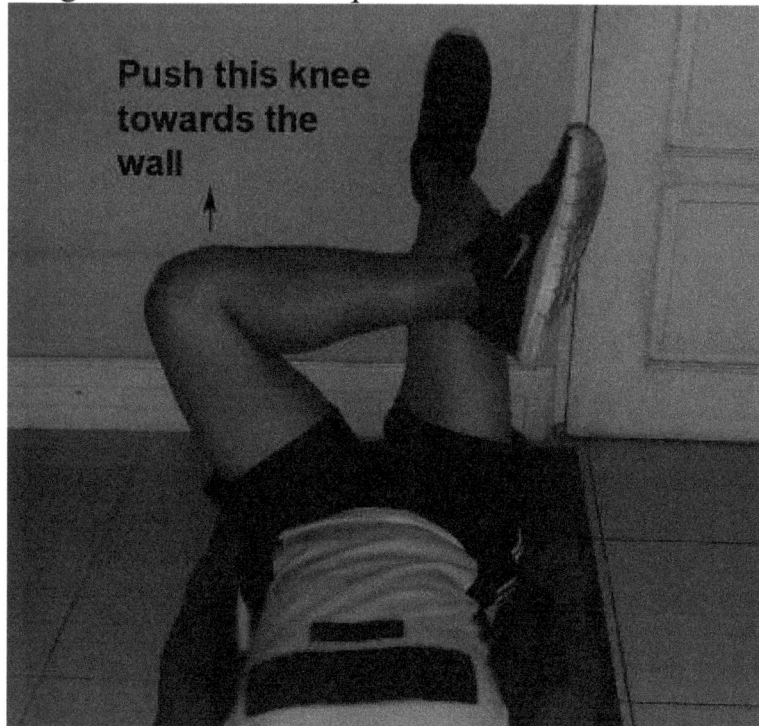

The goal is to get 90 degree angle
on the hips without lifting your butt.
If your butt lifts scoot back

3.) Try to push the knee towards the wall without the use of your hands.
Hold this stretch for 50 seconds.
4.) Do this for both sides.

Standing Hamstring Stretch

This stretch helps you improve the flexibility of the muscles on the back of your upper legs.

1.) Stand erect and raise your arms up.

2.) Slowly lower your arms and reach for the ground

3.) Make sure not to bend your knees.

4.) Keep your hips legs and hands aligned throughout the stretch as shown in the picture:

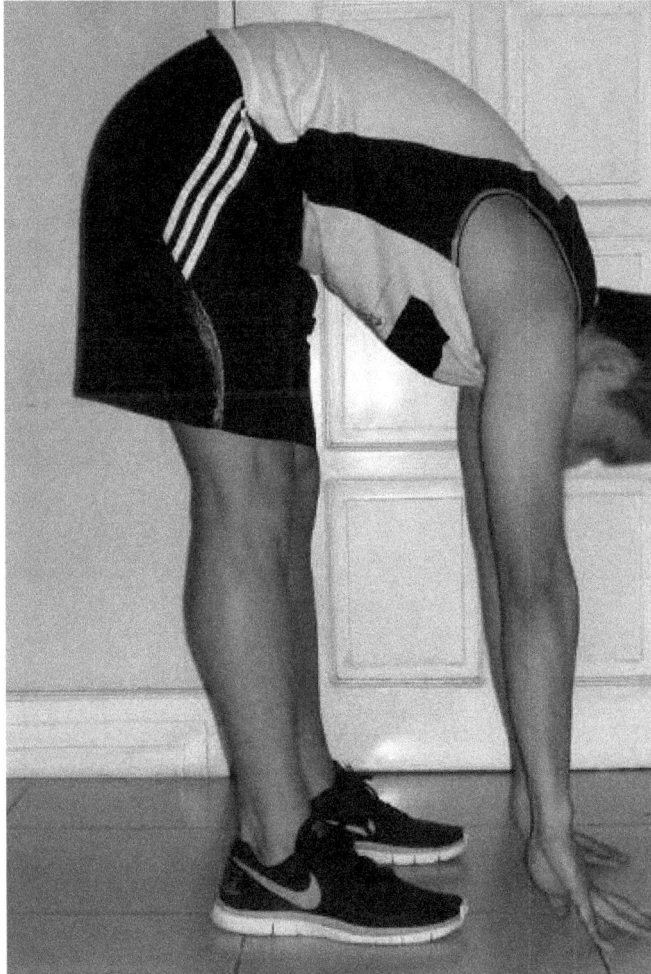

As you get better at it, you can have your palms touch the ground and hold the stretch for 40 sec.

5.) Hold this pose for 30 to 40 sec. As you get better at it, you can have your palms touch the ground.

6.) Remember to take deep breaths.

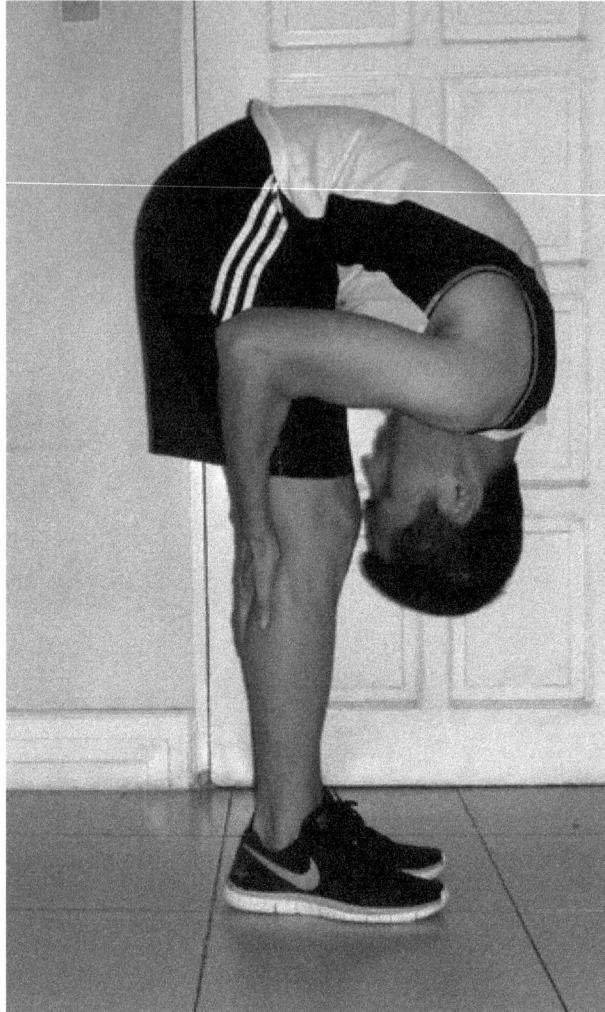

Your final goal is to be able to bring your head all the way down to your knees and hold this stretch for 30 sec.

2. Everymantri, dir. *How to Run Like An Olympian.* Perfs. Joanna Zeiger, Brandon del Campo. *Everymantri,* 2013.
3. *Ibid.*
4. *Ibid.*

Chapter 5

Recruiting the right muscles to improve your speed during propulsion

Another important technique that you should take note of happens during propulsion phase- the part after your foot hits the ground and generates power by pushing off of it.

One of the most noticeable mistakes that you'll find in novice runners is the back-drag. The back-drag is basically the unnecessary and exaggerated push off from the calves as seen in Fig.5B. Notice that a lot of athletes particularly in football and basketball do this a lot. The main reason is that most athletes feel more explosive when they're pushing off the ground using their calves.

While the calves are powerful muscles, using them is very inefficient because it creates an upward force, creating an up-and-down motion for the COG. This leads to mechanical inefficiencies as well. See Fig. 5A.

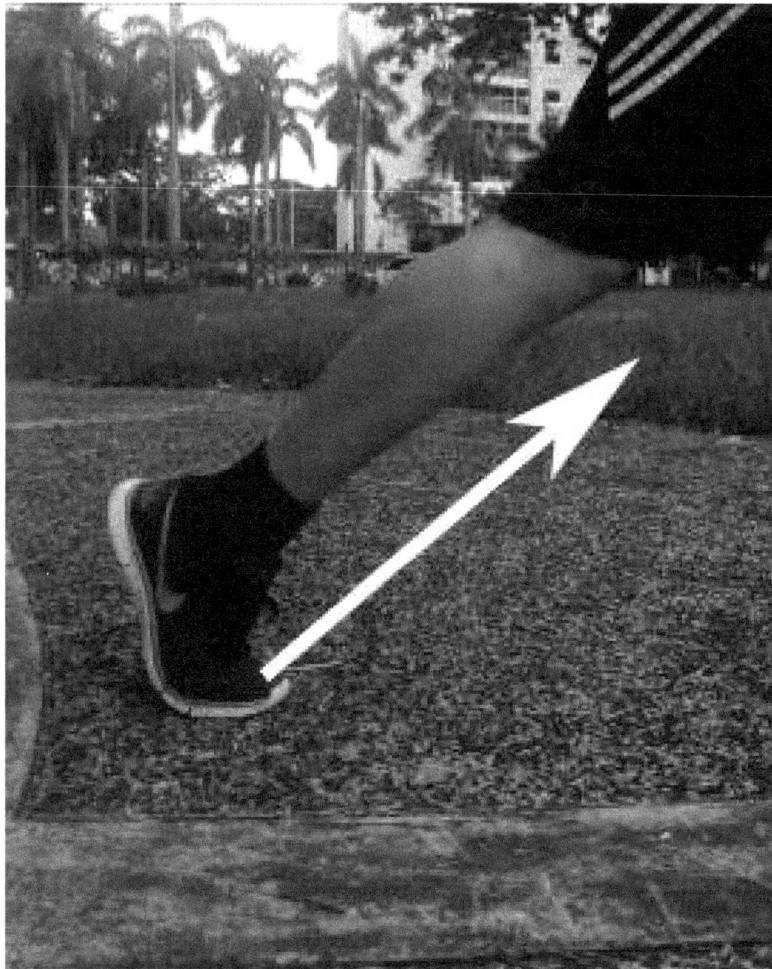

Fig. 5A Exagerrated push off with the calves,
creates a diagonal force that leads to
an up-and-down motion for your COG.

Mistake #7 Exagerrated push-off with the calves after your foot lands

Pushing off the calves also extends your lower limbs far away from your COG and prevents you from using two of the most powerful muscles in your body-your glutes and hamstrings.

The butt and hamstring muscles, being bigger, do a better job of generating force than your calves. (insert source). Moreover, they fatigue less easily which allows you to sustain your speed longer than relying on your calves alone. See Fig. 5B:

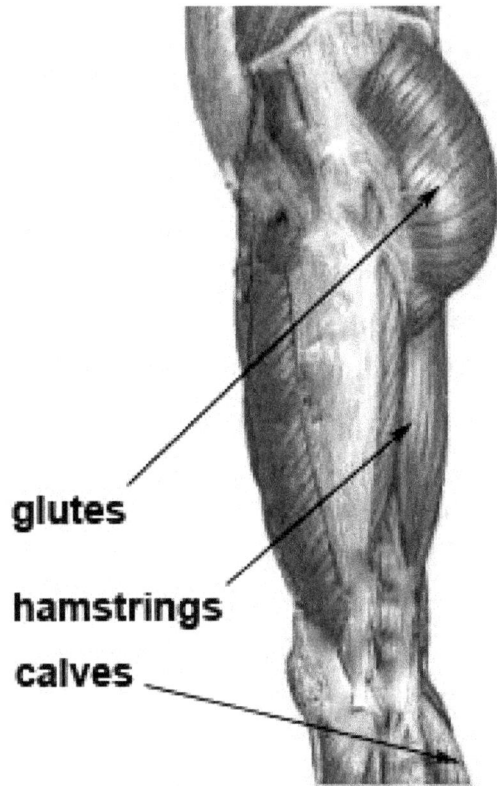

glutes

hamstrings

calves

Fig. 5B Since the hamstrings and glutes are the bigger muscles, they generate far more power pulling the body forward than the calves can at pushing the body forward.

Technique #9
Use your hamstring muscles to generate power to pull you forward.

One of the best ways to get rid of this habit is to use the no-back-drag drill
1.) Lean against the wall and run in place.
2.) Make sure to raise your knees.
3.) You'll notice that the wall stops your lower leg from going too far from your COG.

Your Foot Is Like A Wheel

The wheel is the most efficient way to travel horizontally. If you look at how a wheel of a car travels, you'll notice that the points around the rubber will come into contact with the ground very quickly.

  The same should be true when you're running. You have to minimize the contact time between the ground and your forefoot. Do not wait until your forefoot becomes fully weight bearing.

Technique #10 The contact time between your foot and the ground must be short. Do not wait until the weight has been fully transferred before pulling your foot back.

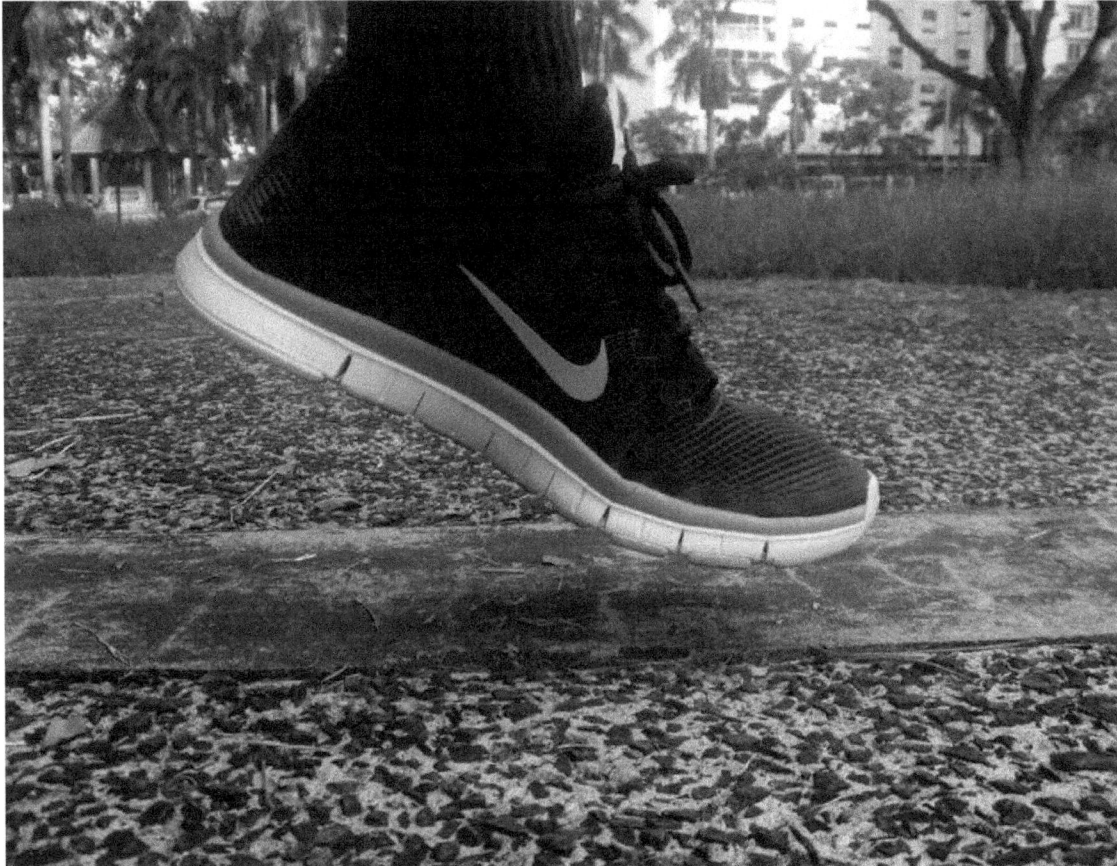

Fig. 5C Think of your foot as a wheel.

Chapter 6

How To Improve Your Endurance

I'm willing to bet that 8 out of 10 beginners will be asking these same questions:

How do I improve my endurance?
When does running become easier?
How come I'm losing my breath after running only a few miles?

The answer to all of these questions boils down to this: correct breathing technique!!!

Now I'm sure most people will read this and ask themselves why they should learn how to breathe properly. After all, breathing is something we've been doing all of our lives, why should we learn to do it at all?

Breathing isn't something that we think about until we've pushed ourselves to our limits and we need to cover the last couple of miles or so.

For most beginners, they usually struggle with their breath trying to get those last few miles because they take shallow breaths. They often tense up and raise their shoulders when they're running.

Although it looks like they're taking in a lot of air, they're not. And they're doing it very inefficiently. To make things worse, they're sucking in their stomach!

So how should runners breathe? The most efficient and effective way to breathe is to do it with the diaphragm. It is only through the diaphragm where you can relax as you breathe deeply and maximize your intake of air. In a few moments, I'll be showing you some drills that you can do to build the muscle memory for deep breathing.

But first, I want you to look at some of the best singers around. They're the best examples of breathing correctly. There is no profession in the world where breathing plays such an important role. Notice how singers take in more air than usual as their belly expands right before they reach high tones. In the same way, your belly should be expanding when you're breathing.

Initially you might struggle with breathing this way at higher intensities but as you get better at it, you should be able to do this easily. The drills below will give you different levels of intensity. Pick one that suits you the most.

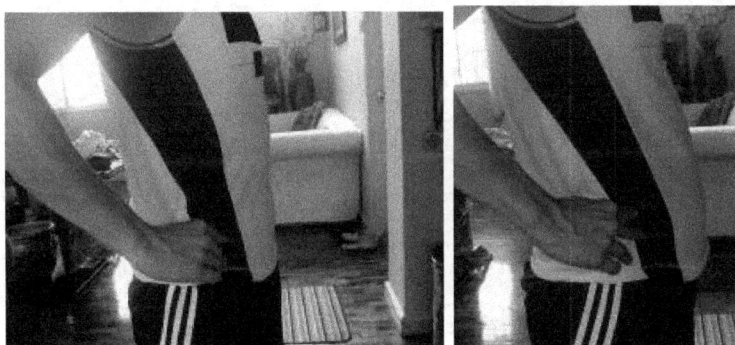

Fig. 6A & 6B You'll know that you're breathing correctly when your belly expands when you breathe.

Here are some drills that I've learned from to help you with your breathing.[5]

Bridge Breathing Drill
1.) Lie flat on your back.
2.) Lift your lower back as shown in the picture below.

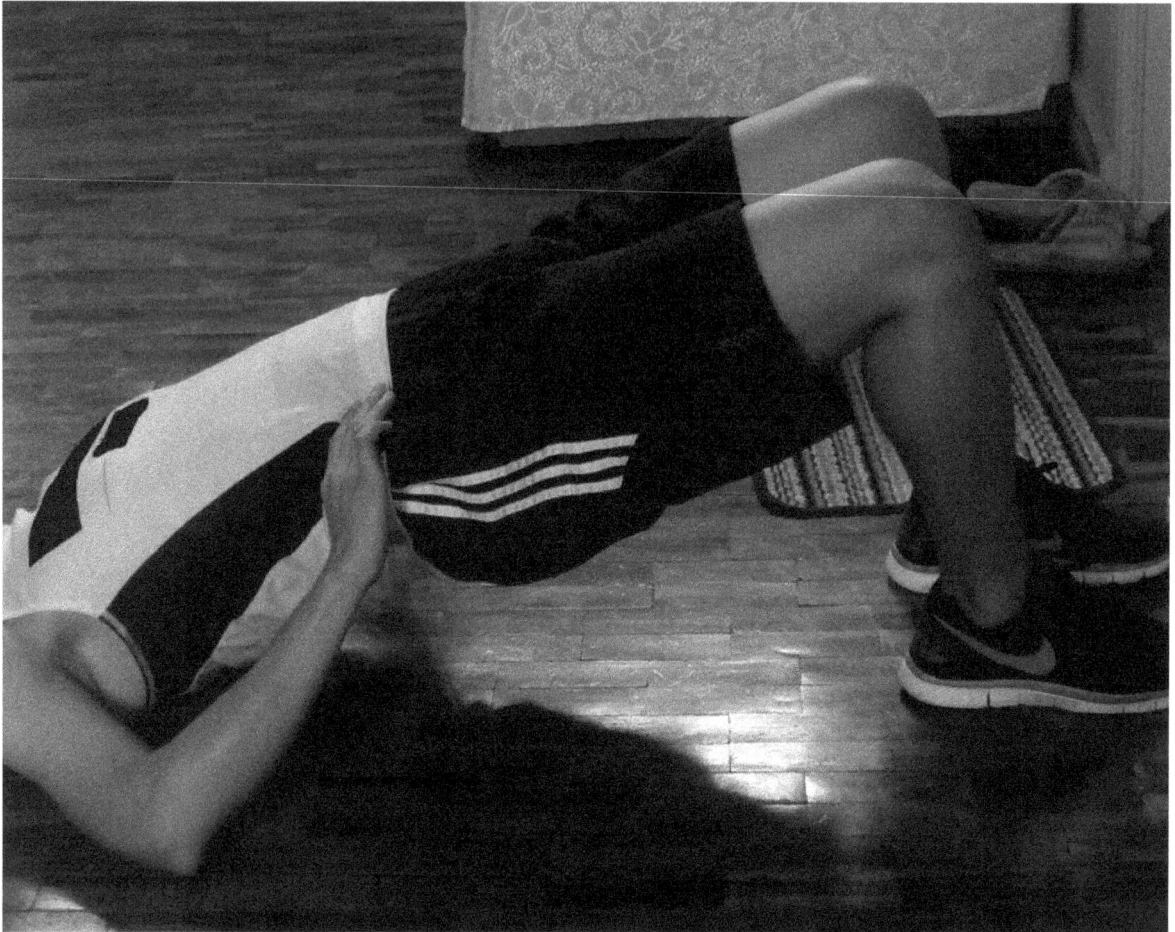

Fig. 6C You should feel a good contraction with your glutes and keep your shoulders flat on the ground.

3.) Breathe from the diaphragm and feel the front and sides of your belly expand.

4.) Hold this for a minute to 2 minutes.

Lying On Your Side Breathing Drill
This drill will help you balance the breathing of both sides of your diaphragm.[6] Normally, one of the sides of our diaphragm is stronger. This drill will be shutting out one side of your diaphragm and opening up the other so you can breathe better on that side of the diaphragm
.

1.) Lie flat on your back with outstretched arms and both knees to one side as shown.

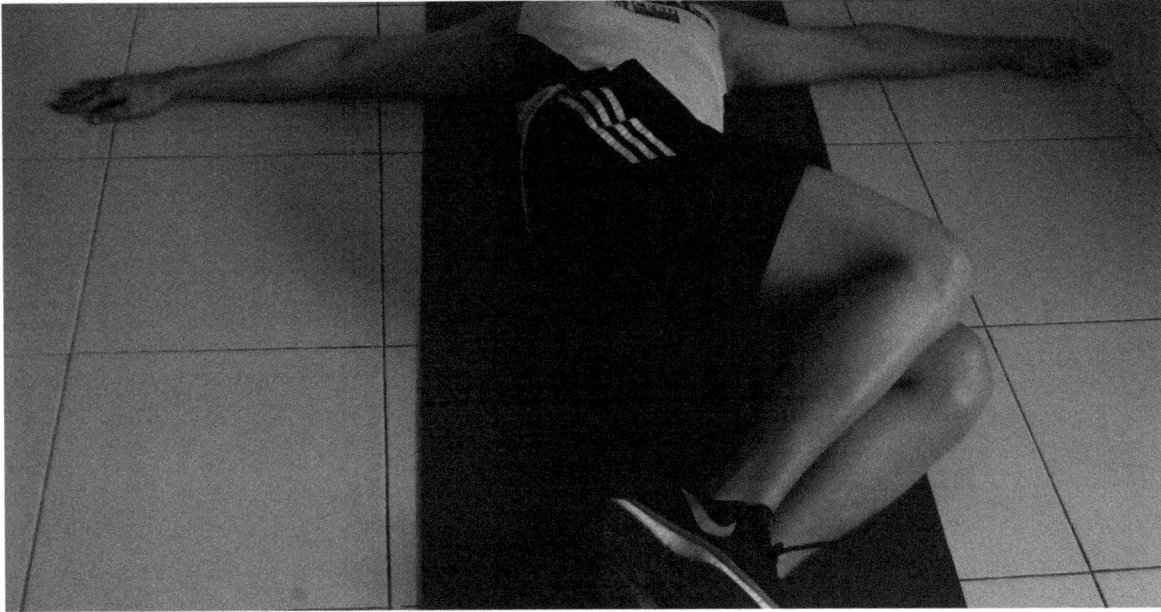

2.) Take deep breaths and do this for a minute.

3.) Do this for the other side.

Breathing Awareness Drill

1.) March in place.

2.) Take deep breaths.

3.) Look at your shoulders. You don't want them rising or having one shoulder up and one down.

4.) Put your pointer finger on the sides of your belly to feel it expand as you breathe.

Core Breathing Drill

1.) Put one foot behind the other.

2.) Take deep breaths with your arms on the sides of your belly while challenging your core.

3.) Do this for one minute.

4.) Switch legs and do the same after a minute.

I cannot emphasize it enough. Breathe through your diaphragm!

Most athletes run out of gas in the late stages of a race. Take deep breaths and expand that stomach with your shoulders relaxed. Don't suck in your stomach the whole time.

5. Everymantri, dir. *How to Run Like An Olympian*. Perfs. Joanna Zeiger, Brandon del Campo. Everymantri, 2013.

Chapter 7

Alignment

One of the things that separates the excellent runners from the rest is their alignment. Any form of side to side movement from your COG doesn't contribute to moving you forward.[6]

Here's what I want you to try out for yourself. Have somebody hold a straight edge vertically and observe the way you run as you run towards him.

If he notices your head, shoulders or the center of gravity move from side to side or vertically that's one of the signs that you're running inefficiently.

Stretches and drills to help your alignment

Posture Analysis Drill [7]
1.) Lie flat on your back.
2.) Make sure your hips are in a neutral position.
3.) Raise your arms and knees as shown in the pictures below:
4.) Do 10-20 reps.
5.) Check for any misalignments. Does your knee, foot or arm tend to go inward or outward when you lift it?

Ankle-knee alignment drill [8]

This drill helps with your ankle and knee alignment when you're running. It also helps with your foot strike.

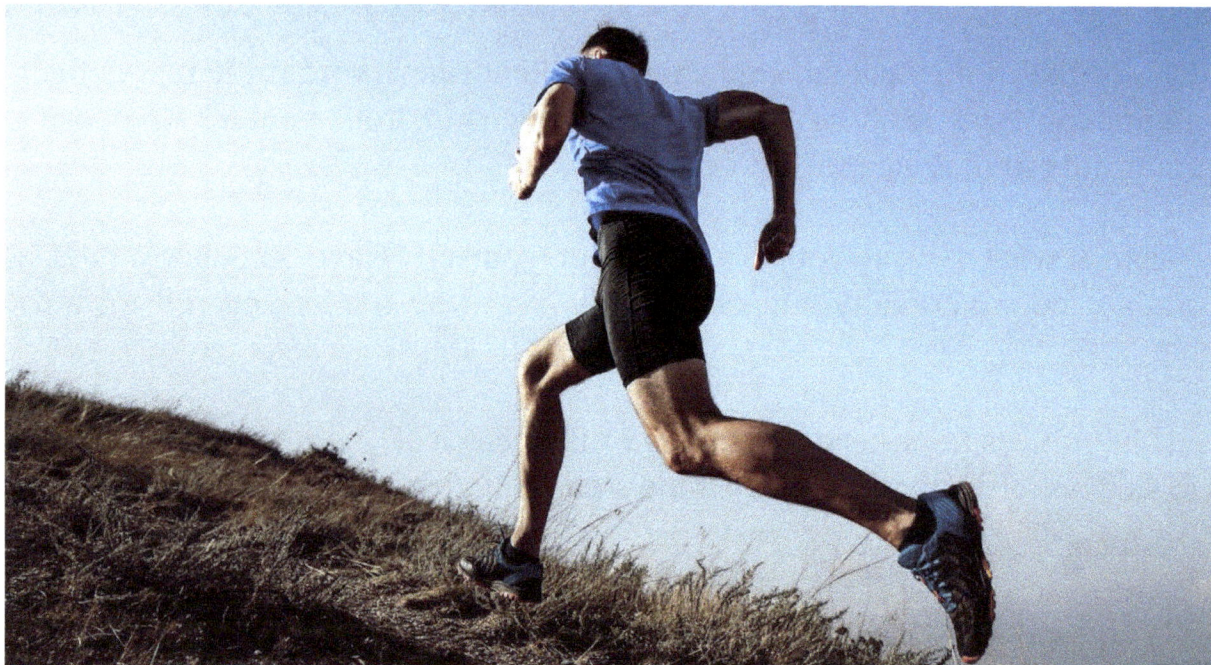

1.) Start with your hips against the bench.
2.) Turn your feet clockwise and counter clockwise rotations for 10 to 40 reps. It may not feel smooth for one side if there's any kind of imbalance.
3.) Flex your ankles forward and back for 10 to 40 reps as shown below.

6. *Human Kinetics, dir. Coaching by the Experts: Track and Field Events. Perfs. Larry Ellis,Stan Huntsman, The Athletic Congress U.S. Track and Field. Human Kinetics, 1993.*
7. *Ibid.*
8. *Ibid.*

Chapter 8

Frequently Asked Questions When Running

When should I do the stretches?

Always warm up for 10 to 12 minutes before doing any kind of stretching. Never do stretches when your muscles are cold. You can always jog in place or better yet do some of the drills in this book to warm up your muscles and increase their elasticity. After you've warmed up start doing the stretches.

Can Running Help Me Lose Weight?

Yes, definitely. In fact most of the experts in weight loss have running as their preferred choice of exercise. Running at low intensity for 30 minutes burns around 180-240 calories.

Remember that running tends to be catabolic (a state where you're losing lean muscle mass). To prevent this, you should be eating enough protein. As a rule of thumb, that means eating at least 1 gram of protein for every pound of weight.

Should I eat before a run? Should I eat carbs before I run? Will that slow down fat loss.

Yes you should eat before a run. Ideally you should eat around 2-3 hours before running.

As for eating carbohydrates before running, that's a bit of a tricky question. For untrained people, fat loss slows down when you eat carbohydrates before going on a run. However, there has been no difference in fat loss between fasting and eating carbohydrates for trained individuals for the first hour and a half of running.

How do I prevent cramps or side stitches?
Side stitches are usually a result of poor breathing techniques, lack of hydration and digestion. Remember to always use your diaphragm to breathe. It's also important to keep yourself hydrated before going on long runs.

One of the most overlooked aspects of getting cramps is digestion. Try to eat a few hours before your runs if ever you get cramps or side stitches. It's very important to listen to your body.

When you do encounter side stitches, slow down to a walk and breathe deeply. Try to keep yourself hydrated as well.

How fast should I be jogging/running?
It largely depends on your training goals. Are you training for a marathon or sprint or fat loss? Are you training for distance or speed or both?

You have to decide what you're going to prioritize. If you're training for speed, you have to improve your form and do sprints from time to time.

If you're training for distance, you might want to go slower and improve your form while doing your tempo runs. The better your form is the more efficient you will be.

If you're training for fat loss, you have to monitor your heart rate. The optimal heart rate for fat loss is the one, which corresponds to 65-70% of your VO2max. You can find calculators for your VO2max online.

What's the best time of the day to run?
The best time to run during the day is any time where you can make it a habit.

For most people, it's in the mornings where they won't be distracted with work and other activities. Others prefer running in the late afternoon after work. Lately, there has been a trend for running at noon.

The most important thing to remember is to turn it into a habit.

Should I run through pain?
That depends on the kind of pain you're experiencing. In general, if you experience any kind of sharp pain you need to stop. If the pain also doesn't go away after a few minutes, you need to stop.

Should I make up the run? What if I miss a day of training?
If you're weeks away from competition, yes you should make up for the missed day.

Can I consume dairy products before a run? Does it cause cramps?
Always listen to your body. If you have any kind of lactose intolerance, don't consume dairy products before your run. Dairy products may worsen your cramps.

What if I have to take a month off from running?
In general, I've noticed that most guys can manage to lessen their running time instead of taking time off.

On the other hand if you're injured and you can't do any running for a month or two, try to see if you can do some of the stretches listed on this book so you can practice and improve on a single area. By the time you start running, you'll definitely start to see some improvements.

Can I Listen to Music When Running?
Do you have to? I strongly recommend against using headphones while you're running.

If you're doing trail-running or on roads, it's best to keep the headphones at home. Dangerous and fatal situations will pop up simply because of a lack of awareness on the runner's part.

Listening to music also hinders kinesthetic awareness, which is crucial when you're trying to improve your running form.

Bibliography:

1. Everymantri, dir. *How to Run Like An Olympian*. Perfs. Joanna Zeiger, Brandon del Campo. Everymantri, 2013.

2. Ish Ledesma, dir. *The POSE Method of Running*. Perfs. Dr. Nicholas Romanov. Ish Ledesma, 2001.

3. Human Kinetics, dir. *Coaching by the Experts: Track and Field Events*. Perfs. Larry Ellis,Stan Huntsman, The Athletic Congress U.S. Track and Field. Human Kinetics, 1993.

4. Ben Landry dir, *Best Running Technique*. Perfs. Ben Landry. Ben Landry, 2011.

5. Eric Feller, dir. *Evolution Running*. Perfs. Ken Mierke, John Bolton. Endurance Films and Fitness Concpets, 2005.

Lightning Source UK Ltd.
Milton Keynes UK
UKHW050843280521
384530UK00002B/250

9 781667 101378